THE SENIOR HOOD STRUGGLING

(To Stay Healthy and Happy)

Diana Harvey Darrisaw

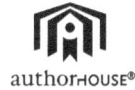

authorHOUSE®

AuthorHouse™
1663 Liberty Drive
Bloomington, IN 47403
www.authorhouse.com
Phone: 1-800-839-8640

First published by AuthorHouse 9/16/2009

ISBN: 978-1-4389-9640-0 (hc)
ISBN: 978-1-4389-9641-7 (sc)

Printed in the United States of America
Bloomington, Indiana

This book is printed on acid-free paper.

Introduction

My name is Diana Darrisaw. I hope we had the pleasure of meeting through my other books, Happy Healthy Seniors and Recipes and Meal Planning for Seniors. I am a retired patient-care food supervisor. Philadelphia is my home. My professional education from Penn State and Georgia State universities prepared me for thirty years as a nationally certified food supervisor. I obtained membership in DMA (Dietary Managers Association) and HFSS (Hospital Food Service Society), two excellent groups fighting for continuing excellence in food service for patient care. Having the chance to work in various healthcare facilities gave me the knowledge of how varied procedures can be, but the ending is the same. Food plays a large part in healthcare, and geriatric care is important and necessary. I am proud to be a part of the blocks that are being used to build a healthier tomorrow for all seniors. Proper medications along with a healthy meal planner are partners in making our days happy and healthy.

Contents

SECTION FIVE

SECTION ONE

What Is The Seniorhood

The seniorhood is the connection from one senior to another all around the world. If you take the time and think about this, you should feel proud. I would like to share my feelings about what being a senior means. A senior should never be in denial of being a senior citizen. Treat the feelings of youth with a wise but long-handled spoon. Looking twenty-five years of age is great, but being a senior and feeling twenty-five is a blessing. There are many who are in denial about their age. Being proud of being a senior can only take place when you can accept it. I only wish it were possible to have a seniorhood awareness organization in every area around the world. What a fabulous legacy we would have and leave for the following generations. Staying connected to each other is important. In doing this we will always be able to communicate with each other and, believe it or not, help one another. Every time someone says or does a good deed in the name of a senior, we all benefit. The following is what a senior means to me ...

S: STRENGTH—In the many battles we have fought in life's struggles.

E: EFFORTS—Always trying to reach a good solid-gold place in our lives.

N: NEVER—Forgetting others in their struggles in life.

I: INVOLVEMENT—Family and friends sharing our needs and uncertainties.

O: OBEDIENCE—Being obedient to our faith.

R: REMEMBERING—The coming generations and their continuing struggles for life's best ...

H: HEALTH—A major necessity in our lives.

O: OPENING—Your heart and compassion to the less fortunate.

O: OFFERING—Solid, helpful information to one another without hesitation.

D: DOMINATE—Our rights that we have as human beings first and seniors second.

If you are not following these steps, start today. When we keep our hopes up and continue our strengths in many areas, it makes it better for all. Let the connection we have with each other be our support and loyalty to one another … Let's use the name seniorhood with pride and determination to do the very best for ourselves. Friends, we must use the storage of words and deeds that we have consumed through the many years of our lives. Work for the good of our senior years. Some of us are going through many private hardships; it touches us all in due time.

Stay Positive In The Most Important Years Of Your Life

Keep a positive focus on life. The years of our lives belongs to us; let's make them mean something. Negativity is just a word; positivity is a word that offers hope. Our grandchildren, other family, and friends are the next generation; we can show them how the battle of health can be fought in a positive way. There are so many of us who are tired from life's toll, and some are just afraid to stand tall for what we know is right. As long as we are alive, we will not be left out of life's surroundings. After all, we are a large part of it. Aging is a process; if you live long enough you will experience all that you need to know. When I was younger, I listened and heard what the older generation was saying. Some topics I followed and understood; others were like the leaves on a windy day, flying by me. Now I am a senior and I do remember what Mom, Dad, and Grandmother said to me. If we continue to have the determination to be heard, hopefully not only will we be recognized, but the seniors who follow will also be. Hold fast to your hopes and dreams. Through some circumstance they can be taken away. Make your late years positive. Sickness is a condition, but hope can be a healer.

Make sure that being able to survive alone is not taken away for selfish reasons by other connecting parties. We have earned these golden and silver years—what other human has the right to take away the preciousness of them? We have raised families; some are still raising families. Ask yourselves when will it be time for me? If you haven't allowed time for yourself, ask yourself why.

Share your continued love with family, but remember that you are number one. To share doesn't mean you go to the back of the room. As long as I am mentally and physically able I will not let anyone take over my thinking or decisions concerning my welfare; only if is for the good. Each generation has a place in this world. All of you out there, give us ours, the seniorhood ...

Stay Focused On Your Medical Team

Illness is something that none of us welcomes. It sometimes takes quite a while to show its face and can last a lifetime. The way we take care of our bodies in the early years plays a large part in what the later years can bring. There are certain situations, such as inherited diseases, which are beyond our control, but a large percentage of our health problems can be attributed to the choices we make. Your medical team is there to assist you and guide you in the right direction for good health. It is important, being the patient, to follow the proper healthcare you have been given. Miracle workers are not found in doctors' offices (smile). Common sense and good directions to better healthcare. Keep your office visit appointments so you can catch a problem before it gets serious.

We as seniors joke around and say we have both feet in the grave and one arm holding us up. (This sounds bad, but if you are a member of the club, you understand the terminology.) Follow your medical directions with sincerity, and do it daily without hesitations. Give your whole body the same care and concern as you would for the new $150 pair of shoes or your new car or the other hobbies and interests that you hold near and dear. Take, as an example, a healthy, green, beautiful plant. If ignored and not cared for it will soon perish; our bodies can be placed in this same group. Each time you miss a doctor's appointment you are the one who is in danger of bad health. A dear friend of mine had a small sore from a prior bruise. It was ignored, and when he did see his doctor about it he almost lost a limb. He had no idea that he had diabetes. Still continuing not to follow the given rules, it wasn't too long before he lost his life. It is no joke; proper healthcare is a must. Let us not ignore the messages our bodies give us when the body is not performing its best. This can happen when you do not visit your doctor regularly and not tell all that needs to be told concerning your well-being. Your medical staff and you make the appointments for your visits, not just you. Keep your appointments for tests and blood work. These are the steps needed to give you the best healthcare possible. When you are prescribed medications, take them as directed, following your prescribed regimen for keeping healthy. Do not use other people's medications, and do not give yours to others. Eat the proper choices of foods. I get so baffled when I talk to someone concerning their illness and they say, "I wasn't told that!" or, "Oh no! I didn't know that." I have worked around patient care for many years, and I definitely know there is no truth in what they are saying.

Each time your medical team has a patient doing well, it gives them time to give another patient who is sick a little more time. The professional caregivers are human like you and I. They have a gift to share, to help others to be as healthy as possible and from this, happiness is a guarantee for nine out of ten patients. Don't change doctors for foolish reasons; I have an associate who has changed doctors three times in one and a half years. Now she has no insurance coverage or doctor.

Your medical staff is not like the latest clothing styles—don't keep changing because you are not allowed to be the doctor. Don't be offensive when you know that the truth is being spoken. We have certain rights and choices. Make sure you use them wisely. I am not tickled pink because I have medications to take daily or a certain regimen to follow for better health. I am no different from any other senior; I have no special powers for better health. I am proud that I try hard every day and make each day the first day of my life. I will accept all that I have to in order to enjoy my golden years. What about you? We must keep that strong, sincere, and honest connection with our medical team in order to have the chance of keeping good health. Walk toward the help you need, not away from it.

SECTION TWO

Be Motivated And Educated In What Your Needs Are

If you have been told that your eating has to change, the first steps are to find a way to become motivated and educated about what your condition is. Make sure you understand your condition and understand what you must look for in your meal planning. This is when you need my H.H.S. (*Happy Healthy Seniors*) beginner's book. It is a small book but a great motivating tool for the beginner in healthy, happy eating. If you have diabetes, cardiovascular conditions, or high blood pressure, go to diabetic classes and check with organizations that will follow up on your health conditions. The American Diabetic Association can offer great help. The American Heart Association can also guide you with your cardiac issues; it is most important to follow your medical advice. With these conditions you must have a solid understanding in order to be able to continue each day on the right foot. Ten out of fifteen people I meet and talk to have diabetes and some sort of heart condition. Learn how to plan your meals with alertness to your NOT needed foods. We must make our meal planning an important link to living a healthy lifestyle. Our lives are depending on it. Family and friends can help if allowed. We as human beings have been given special gifts, two of which are feelings and intuitions. Use them toward your fight for good health and happiness. We have been around a little longer, so we are champs in this area of survival. I cannot put a laugh or smile at every change of thought; I am sure you will feel when the laugh or smile comes in.

Ask questions when you have meetings concerning health matters. Shaking your head concerning certain topics when discussed or written is not enough. You need to take part on a larger scale. When you are away from the meeting, be sure you can relate to what was discussed. When you make your doctor visit, if you are alone, be able to discuss with your family what took place. If you are accompanied by someone, still grasp as much as you can. To educate and to reach for motivation on any given issue that concerns your livelihood is a must and a plus for you. If you have an eating regimen that has been set up just for you in connection with your illnesses, friends, take this tip from me on a serious note: start preparing your own foods at home—get started. We need to know what foods are being used and have an insight into the preparation and cooking. Yes, there are quite a few seniors who are not able, and there are millions who can. Don't let quick and easy be combined with wrong choices in eating. During the summer months I had a lovely lunch out. I felt that I was ordering the correct foods, but the next couple of days, my ankles were puffy. It came from the day's temperature and consuming too much sodium.

We are responsible for all of our needs, and in some way we must see that our health needs are supplied properly. They are many who are ninety years and older and have not stopped trying to supply their needs. My dear mother-in-law is one of the many. She cooks for herself and takes care of all her daily needs. This is how she wants it, and this gives her a purpose every day to push on.

Friends, don't fool yourself: when you become a senior, anything you do that needs the mind or body to make it possible is awesome in a healthy way. There was a time when I had made up my mind that when I reached that precious age of retirement I would not do any more daily cooking or anything else I didn't feel like doing. Well, friends, it all changed. I retired with health conditions. I was sure my vows to myself weren't going to change; after all, I wasn't well. In the course of my struggles I found that activity was one of my best medications.

Seniors, come on. Be real to yourself. You will continue to have health problems if you don't adapt to your given healthy regimen. Make sure ALL your needs are taken care of if you are able. I have a disability, and guess what, friends: I know what I want and I make sure it is done. Reach out and get that extra help you need. Pride is just a name; illnesses you can feel. If your mind is stable, this is all that is needed to make things right for you. If I can do it you sure can too. So you cannot walk or stand; these two things are not needed to extend the mind. Get that wheelchair or motor chair or stool with rollers to work in aiding you in your kitchen. We must be more assertive to our needs. Don't let others discourage you in what you are doing; there isn't any room for negativity. Enjoy the gift of life, and along the way help someone else enjoy it also. Yes, some of us have waited for this time in life to be able to lie back and just do nothing. This can be good and not so good. In order to be a whole person, all of the body must be as healthy as possible, the mind included; we know that the mind is the headquarters for the body.

Associate yourself with people and things that can give you promise, and make your determination to stick to what your goal is. There are exercise clubs out there—check them out. Quite a few exercise programs offer nutrition tips. When we have to make a change and don't know how to get started we need someone or something to help. Don't be ashamed or afraid to discuss a part of your life; others are struggling through illnesses also. Stop being selfish with each other. We all need to grow. Any small or large amount of positive information should be shared. Never listen to the word CANNOT when referring to motivation and education. Make every day a new treasure found for you. Keep in mind that there are many in the younger generation fighting a battle with health issues also. We just happen to have used our bodies longer (smile). Don't hide your hardships. Someone out there can help.

Depression Is Real

Quite a large number of the elderly are mentally and physically tired. All of you out there who are able to keep the mind and body alert, keep up the good work. Certain medications have been said to cause some types of depression. Who can help you with that? Tell your medical staff about any health changes, including depression. I never experienced a lasting depression, but I have loved ones who have. I keep my mind busy getting interested in two hobbies (crocheting and writing). When I am not doing one I am doing the other plus keeping updated about life with family and friends.

Depression and loneliness are causing so many seniors' unhappiness. These days are supposed to be our happy days. The following is a list of symptoms of depression. Check off in your mind the ones that you are battling or have dealt with:

- Out of touch with family and friends
- Hard to give another a smile
- Bitter with everyone for no reason
- House of worship has no interest
- Loss of appetite
- Making up friends and circumstances to fill your lonely days
- Not wanting to accept the aging process
- Remembering the old days and feeling sorry because they are over
- Would rather be alone
- Ignoring phone messages

Friends, the above can be signs of depression. Through the years we have faced many a storm, but we did survive, so let's continue to live as happily as possible. As long as there is a living human there will be hardships and happiness for many.

Talking to family and friends and even strangers can help bring about happiness for you. I myself have sat in the waiting room of various doctors though the years and have met some beautiful people. We all have been blessed with intuition and reflexes.

This is a gift given, and most don't use it for the best. When you meet new people, all of the protection points come out. If you pay attention to your inner feelings it will keep danger from you; it works for me. Don't be afraid to meet a new face. A stranger has made me smile and laugh when the closest person in my life was unable. Fellow seniors, we have to strike outside our circle of family and friends sometimes to get what is needed. This message is not meant to send anyone to go and talk to all types of strangers. This is a message to remind you that everyone unknown to you is not always the enemy. Take great hold of your religious background for the support needed. You can make your own happiness. Never use the word SHAME as a part of your life. We all have won some and lost many, so let your life go on and don't keep looking back to the unpleasantness in your life. Try hard to focus on now and happy tomorrows.

Take full advantage of the senior groups offered. It seems a great place to start. Pick a hobby or two to give you a fulfillment in those empty spaces in the day. I have found that it will give you much pleasure and fulfillment. Check the milestone paper you can find it in any busy area such as in our city of Philly. It offers excellent news covering seniors and coming events, and you may find that it is just what you need. Ours is an awesome senior paper put together by an excellent editorial staff with great coming and going news just for you and me. Look in your libraries, banks, supermarkets, and senior centers get a copy.

Don't sit and wonder. We are not children trying to find our way. Reach out and continue to take hold of life. Some shy away from what is real and some, like myself, don't deny what has been found to be real.

My Introduction To Geriatric Meal Planning

I had no idea that my first job would be my future. In the fifties and sixties it was rough in dietary care. People just were not ready to listen to the new and better discoveries in healthy eating. As the years went by in food service I grabbed all the information I could and stored not only for then but for later in life. I always felt that I would one day be able to express my feelings concerning the nutritional needs of the elderly, and now I am, through my writing. In my early years it was hard to be recognized for good input concerning patient-care food service. You were given a certain boundary, and if you crossed it for whatever reason there was a problem. That ended for me in the later years. I would like to say at this time that we all have someone or something that gave us the extra push we needed to reach our inner satisfaction. I returned to a facility I had left for twenty-five years and returned to a newer, stronger facility. Thanks to you all for allowing me to absorb so much in the field of nutrition in patient care. My last twelve years as a patient-care food supervisor were the best years in food service.

During these years, I had an opportunity to take full responsibility for my work in a professional way. The American Dietetic Association played a very large part in making eating choices better for the patient. Each new dietician and nutritionist brought forth much new and proven information from their sources of education in the field of science and nutrition. I found out as the time went by that the patients only wanted to hear that they were getting better. They were set in their way in terms of food choices. Seniors' illnesses didn't just start; they went back as far as when their lives began. Meal planning does not have to be boring and something to dread. I felt the pain and stress for others for years and learned how to take what I had learned and make eating healthy along with being happy a priority in fighting my health conditions.

My message to my patients was—and now to myself is—that acceptance of what our lives have to be in order to survive is the first sign of strength. To live in a struggle is to be a scholar in the struggle. I found very little to help me adjust to my eating with the illnesses. I looked for compassion, motivation and better human understanding. I finally just reached back and handled my situation in the way I had wanted to help the geriatric patients many years before. After doing this, everything came together for me, and in reading my books it will come together for you. We need the little extra help in how to be eager to change unhealthy habits and turn to fresh and healthy ways in our daily lives. Giving the demand is easy, but what about getting it done?

Fellow seniors, find ways to make the struggle work for you. I feel that there is always a way if sincerity is in place first. Take charge of your meal planning. Make sure your meals have a balance of proteins, fats, and carbohydrates. It does not take fancy food to make meals happy; it takes caring and patience. Why are meals being offered to some seniors daily with three to four starchy foods in one meal and fewer colorful vegetables? I had an opportunity to meet and discuss meal planning with a group of diabetic patients, including family members and friends. They ate a large amount of the time away from home. The excuses they had were, "There was no one but me to cook for; I don't like eating alone; it's easier to call out or eat out." All the reasons fit their lifestyles. My answer to them was that until you take control of your meal planning, the ending process for better health doesn't look too good. Out of the seven people I met with, four have changed their meal planning around for the better and are doing quite well. The other three are continuing on the opposite side of good health; time will tell how they make out. How much is good health worth to you? Think about it. You cooked healthy meals for your family. Did you value your family's health more than your own? Eating for some has no meaning but to fill in an empty spot or to take medications. Eating a large supply of non-nutritive foods can be harmful for you. I was able to take care of patients who appeared very healthy but who had one thing wrong: malnutrition. This condition caused other health problems. I was told that most of them did eat well but the wrong foods. It does matter what you eat for proper health.

Seniors, make that change if this is your lifestyle. If you know someone like this, talk to them and relate what you know; friends share. When some of us had adjusted to the correct way of eating healthy, it was too late. Geriatric nutrition, I have found, needs a lot of time given and a great deal of patience. We, the elderly, are set in our ways, but I have found, by using myself as an example, that if you realize how much of a change is needed, you will become stronger in the fight. Don't be so ready to give up life; it goes fast enough. You will see that special light that is needed for you to find your way; just keep that light burning until you are sure that you have found your way. The introduction I had to geriatric meal planning was long; I learned much and now today use it all to make myself a stronger person and to share with other seniors.

Early Original Food Preparation In Patient Care

As I write, the time comes to mind when almost everything used to assemble a meal tray was done manually. With everything being new to me, I couldn't bear to stand up and cut the large blocks of butter and margarine into small one-serving cubes. Bread had to be bagged one slice at a time. Juice was poured daily, not delivered already portioned out. Diabetic foods were prepared by one cook and one kitchen helper. Each tray was prepared conscious of the correct types of foods and portion control; there was a weighing scale for food at every station. The scales became less and less used through the coming years. There wasn't an area in that huge kitchen where I didn't work in before it was all over for kitchen work for me (after two years).

The next step was passing out trays to patients; it was good because I had a chance to learn and see sickness and understand quite a bit. I am happy that I had the opportunity to have seen and done food-service patient care when I did. I can still now capture and remember the smell of the special rolls and desserts being made for the patients; the special diets were included also, being made a special way. Through my travels in patient food care I always felt more could have been done to give the special diets a wider range of different salads and desserts. I was given permission in my later years to offer special diets—something different but sticking to their diet allowances. It was so satisfying to see their eyes light up with surprise and delight just by my removing and replacing foods. This stuck with me through the years and was a great, great help to me to me in my recipe books. I am happy to say that I made friends with some great professionals and non-professionals in the field of patient care. After five years in the field of food service, I knew what I wanted to do. I started as teen and finished that part of my journey a women.

Patient-care food preparation was done with so much concern and caring, and the rules to follow were a learning tool for many. This information has been offered to let you know that whatever you experience in your lives, if it was good and solid, share it with others. Also, a journey can be hard but fair. Hey out there, if you or your family or friends were in any Philly-neighboring hospital in the sixties up until 2000, I might have had the pleasure of serving you. Let your basketful of experiences and dreams be used to help make a better tomorrow for others and yourself.

H.H.S. Tips and Reminders for Healthy Eating

- Use clean utensils and surfaces when preparing foods (keep away contamination).
- Be careful with knives and food processors.
- It is a must that you eat the serving amounts given for any food's choices.
- Remove the skin on poultry; if you don't, be sure not to eat it when done. Keep your hands washed when handling poultry to avoid food-borne illnesses.
- Purchase dairy products that are low in fats, cholesterol, and salt.
- Grain and sourdough breads are in, and large floury slices are out, for me.
- Make a variety of fruits and vegetables a part of your daily meal planning (fresh is best).
- Frozen vegetables and fruits can be good. After all, they were fresh not too long ago.
- Always keep a variety of foods in your meal planning.
- Kick sodium and sugar, saturated fats, and other unneeded fats and cholesterol (animal fats) to the curb.
- Don't be afraid to try new foods.
- Know what you are looking for on food labels.
- Understand the ingredients used in foods.

In order for any idea or structure to stand strong, the foundation must be made strong. Start your meal planning strong with a determined format for good nutrition, and the daily results will be awesome.

A Cheese Tip

Cheese is one food that can make unhappy foods happy.

The following information can come in handy when deciding to use cheese in various meals.

Processed American sliced sandwich cheese has 105 calories in one ounce and plenty of sodium.

One ounce of low-fat cheddar cheese has 48 calories and sodium and cholesterol.

One ounce of low-fat cottage cheese has less than 20 calories with some sodium.

Calcium is a companion we as seniors need for stronger bones; cheese is made from milk.

- Light cream cheese—a star for calcium
- Parmesan
- Swiss
- Romano
- Monterey Jack
- Gouda
- Asiago

These cheeses are good in calcium. Select low-fat and low-sodium varieties.

Check your store's deli for healthier-style chesses (you will be surprised).

SECTION THREE

Fighting The Battle
Of Diabetes

Diabetes is one of the major conditions that are being struggled with all over the world. All ages are prone to this condition.

Type II (Oral Medications) diabetes is prevalent, with teenagers signing up every day. The media keeps us informed on the rise of both types of this condition.

Type I (Insulin-Dependent) is becoming more and more visible in the elderly. As we all know, diabetes is a disease. I feel comfortable explaining it by using the word condition rather than the word disease. The word disease sounds so incurable and depressing. Take the time to read any information offered to you about the many sides of it. Know exactly what type of diabetes you have (no guessing). Even if you don't have diabetes, having the knowledge of what it is all about may save your life one day. (I am along on this ride, but trying hard every day to get off.) The type is not as important as what you are doing to make it disappear.

How many out there have a good understanding of what part sugar plays in diabetes? I know you have been told over and over; let me explain how I interpret sugars and how they work after entering the body.

Types Of Sugars

Sugar is a carbohydrate; so are fibers and starches. There are three macronutrients that our body needs for daily healthy nourishing. They are carbohydrates, fat, and protein. All three give the body energy and of course calories. There are three types of sugar, and it is necessary to know the role they play once consumed: simple sugar, complex sugar, and alcohol sugar, better known as carbohydrates.

Simple Sugars

Refined sugar is what we place in our sugar bowl. This type of sugar lacks nutrition. There are simple sugars that are natural, found in fruits and dairy products. They do supply nutrition. Sucrose is another name for refined sugar. Simple sugar found in milk is called lactose. If you are lactose-intolerant, your problem appears to be the sugar. The name of the sugar in fruits is fructose. This is classified as natural sugar. We only have control of the amount eaten. This type of sugar can also be found in syrups, jellies and preserves, candies, fruit ices, some sherbets, and many more desserts. Some vegetables carry small amounts of simple sugar. Familiarize yourself with the final three letters of the words on your food labels. If a single ingredient ends with OSE, it is most likely a sugar. Simple sugars digest quickly and can make blood sugar rise swiftly; they also offer quick energy.

Choose simple sugars that will offer nutrition, such as low-fat dairy products and a variety of fresh fruits and vegetables.

Complex Sugar

This is the other sugar and can be found in cereals, breads, pasta, beans, peas, potatoes, cooking flours, a variety of grains, and other starchy foods. It takes these types of food longer to digest because of the fiber content. Simple and complex sugar is broken down inside the body the same, as GLUCOSE the same blood sugar we check when testing.

Alcohol Sugar

This sugar is used in sugar-free products. It gives texture and moisture. Look for this sugar in gum, chocolate candies, cakes, cookies, and other sugar-free products. The name of some alcohol sugars are **Sorbitol, Lactitol, Mannitol, Xylitol,** and **Maltitol**. These sugars are not absorbed completely, and the calories they give are fewer than sugar. Your labels may have these ingredients. Look for the TOL—this will let you know that the ingredient is a type of sugar. Don't pile up on products that contain these sugars thinking that diabetes is not really that strict on sweetness. Too much indulgence in the above will cause elevated sugar. Be conscious of what your choices are at all times. Friends, there are no shortcuts in taking care of diabetes. Check what the FDA has to say about alcohol sugars and artificial sweeteners. The abbreviation GRAS is saying the product is safe. Remember that most simple sugar and alcohol sugar are non nutritive (they supply energy and, calories to the body only).

You have to know ALL the rules with this condition. Check all given information with your health facility. I have found a better understanding in dealing with my diabetes in knowing how different sugars work in the body, and you can too. With medication and a daily proper eating regimen and other good habits we might be able to say goodbye to diabetes one day.

I am not a professional in the field of medicine; nor do I have a master's or bachelor's degree in nutrition. What I do have is the experience of working with patients, one on one, and confronting my diabetes every day. I am using my fight in my condition to motivate you in yours.

We are being educated every day in whatever our sicknesses are. Many of us are looking another way, and some just cannot connect to it all. Please, friends, believe all you are being told by your medical staff and anyone who can give you solid, real, and honest information in your struggle for the best control in your diabetes and any other illnesses. Information is given easily, but being able to accept it is another step, and it can be a hard step. There are many who can adjust to new rules in their diets and ways of life because they never were involved in the style of this particular life. You have to understand all the rules in this condition in order to come out right. Yes, it is a fight, but once you accept it and have the determination to follow the rules, it will become like everything else we must deal with. Only you can make your fight for better health easy or hard.

Through the years I dealt with diabetes with others; it wasn't about me, so my interest didn't focus. Maybe if I had related it to myself as well as I was relating the condition to others, today I might have been diabetes free. Why cry over spilled milk? Wipe it up and keep trying. Waiting until a certain time period to make adjustments is not possible in this department; sudden and quick adjustments are needed. If I wait till next week, or next month, or the end of the year to start my diabetic care regimen, it may be too late for a happy, healthy lifestyle. Don't take that chance. Have patience with yourself and stay positive about getting better. I guarantee that you will, as I have.

Are you checking your blood sugar daily? When I first start testing, I tested three to five times a day until the time came when I knew what foods to avoid as much as possible and what foods to substitute them with and still be able to get the daily needed nutrients in my meals, also keeping my meals happy. If you find that you are having a hard time following the given rules concerning your well-being, you should be talking to your medical staff.

Diabetes is nothing to be ashamed of, only to be dealt with in the correct way. The shame is in not doing your best for your health. Don't continue to do the wrong thing, or the right side will never show. If you are afraid to stick yourself for blood sugar testing or you find that your fingers are too tender to stand the pricking, or if you do not understand what you are reading on the meter or what it means, tell your doctor.

We sometimes have a problem in relating the correct issues to the proper people.

When you don't test your sugar daily, serious problems are waiting for you further down the road. You can be heading for a coma and never know it until it happens. Many are walking around with extremely high blood glucose levels or extremely low levels, both of which can be dangerous. Diabetics are walking around in denial, not being truthful to their medical staff concerning different conditions. They are not willing to believe that the conditions are real and dangerous when not taken care of. Stop doing unnecessary harm to yourself and denying the proper steps you should be taking for a good glucose level. This isn't a game that can be played with your medical team. Why? They know how the game begins and ends.

My trying to have a daily good glucose level is not easy, but it can be done. Think about the hours and days you are adding to your life when your testing comes out where it should be. Make it your aim to have the correct level seven days a week, not two out of seven (smile) ... A lifetime of eating certain foods does not go away easily. Our diabetes conditions vary, but they should all be on the same note, keeping your sugar at the level it should be daily. Friends, one day we will look around and there will be no more insulin or pills to take. Yes, it can happen, and I know for a fact that it does happen. I know that other conditions can develop from poor diabetic management. One illness if not taken care of properly can cause others. I will continue to fight for a healthier tomorrow, hoping you will also. Continue to be assertive to your needs; it does get better in time. Keeping my life precious to me allows me to be determined to fight harder for healthier tomorrows.

We have been around a while, and there isn't very much we have come up against that we couldn't handle. Diabetes will only do to us what we allow. There are things I cannot do anymore, but the mind is still able; this means that the things I want done can still be done. Let your mind control the parts of the body that you cannot tend to any more. After all, the mind is the real force for our thoughts and deeds. Come on, stay determined and strong.

Types Of Artificial Sweeteners

Most likely, if you are diabetic artificial sweeteners is a daily phrase.

The following are non-nutritive and don't offer any calories.

The United States has approved the use of the following, the last time I checked:

- Aspartame
- Saccharin
- Acesulfame-K
- Sucralose

I insist that you check all given information with your medical staff before taking part in any information given through the book. You will feel better (smile).

A Little History

Aspartame is two hundred or more times sweeter than table sugar. This sweetener was approved by the FDA after being evaluated a number of times. It was introduced to me in 1969 as Equal or NutraSweet but was okayed to use in 1981.

Always be informed about what is available as a sweetener and get some solid information on the product. My first choice of a sweetener wasn't good; I kept getting headaches.

Sucralose is about six hundred times sweeter than regular sugar. This sweetener is not absorbed well and was approved by the FDA in 1998. It is used in a number of desserts and beverages and can be used with heat, in baking, and in regular cooking.

Saccharin has been around for decades and is about three hundred times sweeter than regular sugar. It was approved in 1991. There is only a certain amount allowed in foods, and it should be on the labeling. It can be used in cooking. Sweet'N Low is the trade name.

Acesulfame-K is two hundred times sweeter than sugar. The K stands for potassium. It was approved in 1988. This sweetener can be found in baked goods and soft drinks. There are some table-top sweeteners, such as Sweet one.

Sunette is one of the brand names used for this sweetener. This is a fairly new product to me.

HHS Tip

There is a sweetener called Maltodextrin. It is derived from Potato, rice, and corn starches. Check your supermarkets and other stores that carry sweeteners to find out more.

Grandparents, if you use artificial sweeteners in your drinks or foods, make some with regular sugar or honey for the grandkids. They still need the calories. Artificial sweeteners were made without children in mind.

Food Choices For Diabetic Meals

Incorrect Food Choices
Use the following information as a guideline:

- Oversized servings of meats and meat substitutes. Fatty meats that offer high fat and cholesterol.
- Starch—planning meals with three to four starches in one meal
- Vegetables—cooked in fatty substances. Using vegetables in the bread group with other starchy foods (peas, corn, winter squash, and pumpkin) and more.
- Dairy products high in saturated fats, trans fats, and other unhealthy fats, and also cholesterol. Overloading simple and alcohol sugar.
- Desserts—Syrupy canned and jarred fruits. Pies, cakes, and cookies overloaded with simple, complex, and alcohol sugars. Over-large portions of fresh fruits.

Correct Food Choices
Use the following information as a guideline:

- Lean meats and healthy choices of meat substitutes. Remove skin and extra fat from meats.
- Starch—choose a variety, following the given allowances.
- Vegetables—eat as many as allowed (a variety of green leafy veggies, and also veggies with assorted colors).
- Fats—read labels well for low amounts of saturated fats and trans-fats. Keep the cholesterol level to zero or low. Don't aim for high sodium.
- Dairy foods—low in fats, sugar, sodium, and cholesterol.

- Fruits fresh or unsweetened canned. Low-calorie desserts. Keep portion control in mind at all times.
- Use an artificial sweetener if needed.
- Make milk a part of your daily meals, if it is a part of your diet. (Stop skipping around this almost perfect food.) Make the use of an assortment of flavorings to make your milk happy with taste.

You can get examples in my book on recipes and meal planning.

Choose all food products for need first and pleasure second. Most of us do the opposite. I was among that group, but time taught me different. I am glad I had the time to make it right.

Don't go half the way with your condition; you have to be committed to go all the way.

We must take what we have and turn it around to a blessing; friends, we have a chance to do better in our fight.

How many didn't have the chance to fight for health? I can name plenty.

Always keep in good connection with your medical staff; this is the necessary key to open the doors for better health.

Turning in the direction of medical care, you will read often through happy, healthy seniors' books that there are many who haven't followed this rule through the struggle, and they wonder why the struggle hasn't become less. We can be our worst holdback for better days.

We are at the age of life when we are familiar with all the bad and good punches life offers.

Fellow seniors, I am talking to you from one adult to another. Life is offering all the seniorhood to come aboard for a long, long ride on a health cruise, with the final stop being happiness and a healthier you. I was one of the first to pick up a round-trip ticket.

Join me. It will be a happy and healthy ride.

H.H.S. Tip
Sugar is not the only enemy in diabetes.

The Importance Of Reading Food Labeling

Nutritional Facts and Ingredients

You have a food-related illness and have been instructed how much sodium, sugar, fats, and cholesterol to consume. You must understand what you will be reading on food labeling and ingredients. How does what you read connect to what is good for you? The information from nutritional facts helps to keep you at the correct sugar, calorie, sodium, and fat levels. You can never have too many measuring charts or information on the contents of the foods eaten. Keep needed information concerning good meal planning in the prep area of your kitchen. The following are some wordings that you will find on food labeling:

mg: a milligram is a thousandth of a gram.
g: 30 grams is =30 cc. and for dry measure is 1 ounce
K: potassium
NA: sodium

If you are allowed 1,000 cc of liquids in one day and you consume only three eight-ounces portions of liquids that day, you have consumed all together 720 cc of fluids. You have 280 cc more to have before bed as a snack such as Jell-O, fruit ice, sherbet, or milk.

How did I come up with that? The following will show how your 1,000 cc of fluid was used.

A glass that holds 8 fluid ounces x 30 cc = 240 ounces

You drank three eight-ounce glasses of liquids, and 3 x 240 = 720 ounces, so there is 280 cc left.

1000 - 720 = 280cc

If your health regimen includes you keeping your fluids low, this information will be a plus to know. I found it to be great. It you find it to be confusing, pass it up until you can comprehend it much better. Continue to do it your way if it is working for you. Any food that starts as a liquid has to be counted as a liquid, such as Jell-O, ice cream, water ice, or sherbets.

If you are allowed seven servings of meat or meat substitute a day, you will have eaten in grams seven ounces of meat.

How does all of the above connect to how much is good for me?

It connects 100 percent if you are a diabetic or a cardiac patient or both. How much you consume in foods and liquids is a constant red light ON. Your medical staff can inform you better than anyone else how it all connects. For me, it is the connection I need to keep living.

Friends, the danger is that the majority of us will not eat only a serving.

If you purchase a product that gives seven servings and offers 30 mg of sodium per serving, the package as a whole consists of 210 mg of sodium. How many of us will eat one serving? It is time again to practice your multiplication table (smile).The more we eat, the higher all the nutrition facts get. A favorite phrase of mine is portion control. Yes, it is a very hard phrase for a food lover to use, but keep trying.

Always store what you learn in your mind or make a notation of it to refer to at a later time. This can save you stress and the beginning of a possible mild depression (smile). How many times have I said that I can't remember something I was just told? Sound familiar? All forgetfulness is not the big A ...

Ingredients also play an important part in reading food labels. Knowing what is in a product is necessary. There are unfamiliar words being used, and becoming familiar with them allows me to keep my allowed and un-allowed foods in the correct perspective. Through reading different sections of this book, different wordings to look out for on your ingredients' labels will be noted.

There are many myths concerning diabetes. Be sure you recognize the truth.

Have you heard these facts/myths before?

1. Too much sugar causes diabetes. True or false

2. Read your glucose daily. True or False
3. Genetics, overweight, age, and certain illnesses have no bearing on a being diabetic. True or False
4. Foods, candy, ice cream, soda, and salty foods alone cause diabetes. True or False
5. Asking questions, reading information, attending seminars, and diabetic classes will not help. True or False
6. Diabetes has nothing to do with the pancreas. True or False
7. Don't eat simple or complex sugars and diabetes will disappear. True or False
8. Eat whatever you choice and take your medication and your blood sugar will be just fine. True or False.
9. When you eat the wrong foods, double your medication. True or False
10. Obesity is not a danger for the diabetic. True or False.
11. All artificial sweeteners offer good energy. True or False
12. Taking your blood sugar is not important. True or False
13. Using regular sugar is all right; it will not raise your blood sugar much. True or False
14. Eat your meals at a different time every day. True or False
15. Cookies are all right to eat for a diabetic as long as they have no icing. True or False

Further in the book the correct answers await you ...

There is no crime in falling back to not eating properly. The crime is the continuation when **the doctor has told you that your glucose is out of whack and you do have diabetes. Stop the denial approach; the longer you take to get on board to a better glucose level the harder for you.** The following information is worth looking into.

Removing And Replacing Foods

Many years ago I was introduced to the **EXCHANGE SYSTEM** in meal planning for diabetics by the American Diabetes Association (ADA), which I felt was the most spectacular system for happier eating that could ever come about. The name of my system I have used for years is **REMOVAL** and **REPLACEMENT**. These two names were chosen by me because they felt comfortable. Both systems give the person an opportunity to be able to move their foods around at times and replace one food for another in the same food group.

If you are diabetic I am sure the exchange system has been introduced to you. We all follow removal and replacement in my family; it has been proven to be a good thing. Don't remove nutritional foods for less-nutritional foods. If you stay within the same food groups, your calories will stay the same.

Vegetables are one of many important sources for obtaining good nutrition. How much do we understand about vegetables? Are peas, green lima beans, corn, winter squash, taro root, and turnip bulbs vegetables? Some say yes, and references say no. These foods contain enough starch to be listed with the starchy foods such as rice, bread, grits, and pasta. The color doesn't always signify what group a food is in. The bright colors of these foods tell quite a few people that this is a vegetable and I can eat as much as I want. Remember that the vegetables that you have been allowed to have often carry some calories also.

What is needed in deciding on your meals is the best knowledge possible concerning the foods you are going to be using. You cannot shop, prep, or cook your foods with the same old intentions. You have to remove the fatty and salty meats used for seasonings. Get rid of the highly saturated butters, oils, and cooking sprays. Use fresh garlic or garlic powder, not garlic salt; use more of your favorite spices or an assortment of flavorful herbs. Peas do supply some protein. Don't use peas as a meat substitute; adding other protein foods to make up the proper amount of protein needed is a good move.

Since I am on the subject of protein, too much protein can cause a problem when you have diabetes. How many times have we eaten peas and corn, green lima beans and corn, rice and corn, potatoes and peas, or pasta and corn? There are many variations of starch-on-top-of-starch meal planners.

Remember that foods just looking good is not one of the important landmarks for the diabetic. What about holiday time? It is so hard. You can have the same regular meal, turned around to fit your lifestyle; I haven't missed out on any apple pie, tasty sweet potatoes, or macaroni and cheese. It all can be found in my book (*Recipes and Meal Planning for Seniors*). Whatever we eat has to be guided by portion allowances. Keeping the same positive eating regimen has to be done even at these special times. Never attempt to use the exchange system or my system without consulting your nutritionist or dietician. (I have had mixed feelings on how dietician should be spelled. Webster gives two choices; the above is mine.)

Self-assurance is something that can only be sustained by you ...

Know Your Safe Areas
(Mr. B. And Mrs. J.)

Each diabetic patient's calorie needs are different. The amount of calories you are given to plan your meals by is to me just like a medication that has been prescribed. Friends, don't be afraid to ask questions when it is necessary. The safe areas in what you should or shouldn't do are a must to know. There is no room for shyness or ignorance when it comes to your wellness. Some might say that I worked with it so of course I would know. So true, but I live it every day also. Persistence in following your given rules is the ammunition needed to help fight diabetes.

Do not change your medications and meals around constantly; you are confusing all the parts of the inner body like blood, organs, cells, and other parts that help us to stay maintained. I can hear the various parts of my body saying, "What is going on? I needed that medication hours ago," or, "I am tired of the same fuel," meaning foods. It might read funny, but it is very true. Think of your inner body as exactly what it is—you.

If you have diabetes and can't understand why because you always ate healthy, this is something to discuss with your health team. Keep in mind that your family tree plays a large role in some aspects of your health. Let's not be angry at ourselves or others because of what our responsibilities are. Let meal time be a happy time, along with healthy. We are able to turn any bad thing around if we try. There are certain foods we crave, and because they have been restricted we have a stronger desire (smile).

If you enjoy eating the rich cooked foods that offer butter, heavy cream, syrupy sweet desserts, and pastry to die for, this is not a wrong desire. It just makes it harder knowing that you are unable to have it; being a diabetic can be depressing if allowed. Good meal planning can turn any food-related illness from black to a bright sunny color. There are quite a few myths concerning various illnesses; this is why a professional should be the one you talk to. Medically you can be guided, but you have to do the controlling. I would like to share a short story of two patients with similar health problems, but each accepted them in a very different way.

Mr. B.'s and Mrs. J.'s Diets

In my early years as a supervisor in patient-care food service I was given two patients. Mr. B. was a large built man, with his own stubborn ways; he wanted to eat without changing. He was pleasant to talk with and a senior. When admitted he was put on a 2,000 calorie diet. Mrs. J. was a small quiet lady, also a senior, and was admitted with a history of diabetes and cardiac problems and put on an 1,800 calorie diabetic, 2,000 milligram NA (low sodium) diet. Mr. B. was a man with a tremendous appetite and was used to eating whatever and whenever. My first intentions to turn his eating habits around were quite a battle. He needed to become a more disciplined person in his meal planning. His stay was two weeks. Before he was discharged I gave him a diet consultation, short but to the point. He was willing to follow the given rules in his meal planning.

He kept up with appointments, staying the same in weight and glucose levels. He did try very hard, and it started to show in his follow-ups. My other patient, Mrs. J, was a poor eater. The foods she was crazy for were deli sandwiches, salty snacks, candy, and cookies. She couldn't pull herself away from regular soda, by the cans. She stayed for three weeks and had snacks coming into her faster then we could catch them. We had to ask nursing to lend us their eyes for a while (smile). After constantly coming back as an inpatient for the same illness, in between visits she obtained an infection. She missed some appointment for checkups and was not following the proper boundaries given by her medical staff or nutritionist, Mrs. J, sorry to say, had to have a limb removed. A sad but true story.

Take your medications, and you must eat properly also. Stop, stop not taking your blood sugar. I have to say more on this very serious part of healthy diabetes (you and your blood meter). So many are not testing their blood and are determined not to. This is so unsafe. I have found that the majority don't test because they know they are not on the correct eating regimen. To actually see a three-hundred or four-hundred meter reading is frightening, but they are still not ready to leave the cheesecake, to stop overloading on potatoes and rice, and to avoid tons of fast foods daily when out, snacking through the day on high-sugar foods. Make it a daily practice to take your own glucose levels; it can save your life one day.

Depend on yourself as much as possible.

We all have those days when we are spoiled by a spouse or children, or even grandchildren (I do). But diabetes is something we have to take charge of ourselves if able. Friends and associates tell me often that their husband, son, or grandchild pricks them for their blood testing. Find something else to be spoiled with. The more you test yourself the stronger you become in getting that small amount of blood (smile). The majority of us have been afraid, and some still are. Just say to yourself either I will live the best life possible or I'll just exist with no hope or love of oneself. Believe me you will start sticking to get blood (smile). If you have a friend or family member, ask them how they feel about taking their blood sugar. You may be surprised that someone might have felt the same way you do at one time or another. It will make a stronger you. I test two to three times a day. Believe me, I am not crazy about it, but it has to be done in order to follow my meals properly. If my reading is 120, at the next meal something non-nutritive or low in nutrition will be removed. But like everything concerning your health, talk it over with the professionals. Read well what I am saying for motivation; remember this is all about me … We all are different although our illnesses might be in the same circle. Testing is not to be ignored for two and three days at a time. What about the person who states, "If

I don't eat I do not test, or if I have eaten too much I know my sugar is up; it will upset me if I test." Friend, it will hurt even more not knowing and being unable to help yourself.

Stop shying away from what a large amount of seniors are doing (not wanting anyone to know they have a condition, keeping health secrets that may cause them their life one day). I am told often, "You don't mind discussing your illnesses. Why should I? It is not going to make them go away." I don't shout from the rooftops, but I am not ashamed of my health. I am just trying to make it better. I have vanity in myself as a person, not just in one area of my life. Diabetes is a condition for me, and any condition can be fought. I was told as a child that hidden secrets never stay hidden.

As parents and grandparents, let's encourage the youth. They must start at an early age to eat healthy to avoid possible illnesses later.

ANSWERS TO DIABETIC FACTS/MYTHS

1. False
2. True
3. False
4. False
5. False
6. False
7. False
8. False
9. False
10. False
11. False
12. False. A good question to discuss with your medical staff.
13. False
14. False
15. False

Hope your score was a high one.

SECTION FOUR

Fighting For A Better Heart (Cardiovascular Conditions)

The heart is the center of life. When something goes against the way nature has arranged for the heart to respond, this can mean serious trouble. Food is also life. So here is another connection to cardiovascular conditions and food. Sodium is one of the enemies of this condition ... Some of us were introduced to salt at a very early age. The first spoon of table food was probably from Mom's or Grandmom's plate, right? This was the beginning of the use of salt (sodium). Salt does enhance the flavor of foods, but it can easily become an addiction for some. There was a time when certain foods had no attention from me unless I had salt to add. Most of my associates who don't over-indulge in sugar and salt were not allowed to eat either one to the extreme at a young age. The need for certain things to make our lives more pleasant comes under the heading of desires. The indulging in candy and salty snacks was done mostly outside of the home in my growing-up years.

Any food that is labeled rich and gourmet is a mouth-watering invitation. I once was in this line of food choices. I am unable to eat it anymore and haven't been able to for quite a while. If you are in no danger of any food-related illnesses, enjoy, beware, and stay alert, because overindulging might make you my partner in healthy meal planning ...

Fats And Cholesterol Are Different

Fats and cholesterol are needed to stabilize continued good health, as much as other components. There are good fats and bad fats. Any type of fat will cause weight gain. Dietary fats come in a variety of forms. Triglyceride is a form of fat in foods and the blood. Other forms are trans fatty acids and saturated, polyunsaturated, and monounsaturated fats. Margarine is a sample of trans fat. When unsaturated fat goes through hydrogenation, the results are trans fatty acids. The body uses this fat just like saturated fat, and it can be harmful. Beware of foods that have been hydrogenated. Stick margarine is an example. Fats are needed in the body to perform very important functions, such as carry, absorb, and store the vitamins A, D, E, and K in the bloodstream. Fat is stored in the fat cells of the body for later use. Fat is a pillow of protection for organs and also protect them from injuries. Body temperature is regulated with fat. So you see the importance of fat. When you have high levels of bad fat circulating in the body, it is looking to start trouble. It will build up and start attaching to the walls of the arteries that supply blood to the heart and brain ... We don't need a stroke just because we didn't care enough to plan healthier meals and couldn't resist the many cookies, cakes, pies, French fries, and burgers that were cooked in improper (hydrogenated) oils.

Cholesterol has its own duties to perform in the body. This substance doesn't supply energy to the body, because it carries no calories. Cholesterol isn't a fat; it is a waxy substance found in the blood and tissue. This substance is discussed along with bad fats because they are partners in crime. There is no need for extra cholesterol. Our bodies manufacture their own cholesterol.

I have to take caution in my cholesterol consumption daily. It is another red flag for me. Believe me, very little cholesterol from outside the body is let in.

All three (saturated fat, trans fats, and triglycerides) cause cholesterol to rise. When you eat large amount of dietary cholesterol, you are adding more to what you have, and you are ready for medications to help keep things regulated. Just because you are getting help for a better cholesterol reading this doesn't mean it is all right to eat as much cholesterol food as you want. Seniors, the topics and opinions that are being given may appear to you to be unreal, but take it from me, the supplier, they are very real. I am talking and researching based on others' opinions, and of course my personal experience is being used. This way the reality of my sharing can be truly felt. If you want a fairy tale told, sorry, this is the wrong book. This is the route I have chosen to connect with all of you. If you as the reader look at your health in an honest way,,then some of these topics may apply to you..

I found that after cutting way back on extra-cholesterol foods and continuing to take my medication I have had great cholesterol medical reports. It wasn't a drastic step to take, just common sense. If you don't consume the cholesterol and bad fats, you have to be a winner in time. I will not lead you to believe I am free from salt, sugars, bad fats, and cholesterol. I make my desired food choices with a concern for moderation and use portion control 85 percent of the time with my meals. I am not the miracle lady for eating healthy. I am a senior trying hard every day to be healthy and happy and being real to my cause. I am human with desires and needed pleasures in food. I enjoy a variety of foods within limits: seafood, cheesecakes, strawberry shortcake, and plenty of butter and sour cream on my baked spuds (potatoes). My battle started many years ago, when food was my field of work. I didn't take time to listen to all of the warnings. Now as a senior I have to accept the outcome but don't have to accept it without putting up a fight for a healthier me.

I practice daily to keep it all together following my meal-planning regimen. The key word to it all is to try.

H.H.S. Tip

When you purchase dairy foods and other foods that carry fats and cholesterol, remember that you want to see beside each nutritional fact a low number (one to two, or none). This I have found is the safe way to read nutritional labels.

I found that the danger of cholesterol is the amount eaten.

What Is Sodium?

Sodium chloride is the name for the white crystals that some use to an extreme in our food preparation and after the meal is on the table. Yes, good old salt. Sodium is a mineral that many compounds arise from. Salt is only one of the many compounds that come from the mineral sodium. If you have a sodium restriction and are watching out for sodium contents in foods, you have quite a bit of reading in store. The ingredient labels on your food purchases are the place to start. The following are types of sodium you can find on food packages and cans and boxes.

- Baking powder
- Worcestershire sauce
- Monosodium glutamate (MSG)
- Baking soda
- Soy sauce
- Teriyaki sauce
- Sodium benzoate
- Caseinate
- Nitrite
- Sulfite
- Sodium chloride (table salt)
- Kosher salt, sea salt, and gray salt

Friends, sodium is sodium. There is much solid information on the category of sodium, an important mineral. Always search and ask questions concerning what you have been restricted on. You have to be your own investor and protector in your health, like so many others are.

When a food is not sodium free, this information should appear on the nutritional fact panel. I understand that a food product that exceeds 360 mg Na per serving cannot be classified as a healthy product. A food product that offers a meal should not exceed 480 mg Na per serving to be classified healthy. This is my understanding, and I base my choices on this information. Do some checking for yourself.

If sodium is a danger to you, knowing as much as possible can help save your life. Get some use out of your computer beside the chat rooms (yes, I know all about them; some good conversations are going on). Go online to Google to find out about types of salt. Take advantage of the free reading materials offered by companies and various associations. There are a lot of us who cannot get out and around anymore, so contact by phone or mail different organizations that have been set up just for seniors. **Ask questions.** Stop holding back from possible help.

Levels Of Sodium In Various Foods

All foods carry sodium, even fresh foods. When you eat low-salt foods beware of how much you consume. If the food that is low in salt is eaten enough, believe me it will have a high total. If a product with 30 mg NA per serving is eaten three times in one day, you will have eaten 90 mg of sodium. If you eat the same amount of that product for the next two days, you will eat 270 mg of sodium. This is why it is not always what you eat but how much. Keep in mind that this is not the only food you will probably eat, so your sodium intake can easily go past your limit.

The following is an example of how fast a medium amount of food can raise your sodium. A meal can be healthy if not planned correctly unhealthy.

Diana's Meals (2,000 mg NA Allowance per Day)

BREAKFAST
½ cup oatmeal—2 mg Na
1 egg (medium)—55 mg Na
3 fresh apricots—2 mg Na
1 cup flavored (vanilla) skim milk—126 mg Na
Decaf hot beverage
Total Sodium—185 mg Na

LUNCH
3 ounces baked chicken—63 mg NA
1 cup fresh cooked beets—484 mg NA
1 medium baked potato—10 mg NA
Tossed green salad with low-salt dressing—30 mg NA
1 cup skim milk—126 mg NA
1/4 slice or ½ cup cubed cantaloupe—12 mg NA
Snack: small fresh apple—none
Total sodium for meals—725 mg sodium
Amount sodium eaten so far—910 mg NA

Let's see how well you can finish the rest of the meals for the day. It should be a breeze; you have a little over 1,000 mg of sodium to work with. You even have enough for a snack before bed.

Friends, I have to remind you not to try anything different in your meal planning without checking with your medical staff.

Three meals plus snacks can add up pretty fast, even if you choose your foods following the correct rules. I prefer to eat small meals (six per day including my snacks); this is not advice to follow if you have diabetes without checking with your nutritionist. Be patient and obedient in what you are striving for and all will be good. Make sure your favorite vegetable does not include a large amount of sodium, like my favorite, beets. The amount is also necessary to keep in mind if you have problems with sugar.

Do you know that one cup of fresh cooked beets has over four hundred mg NA and about sixty to seventy-five grams of sugar? I do know how to pick the rich choices (smile). Many of us do not realize how sodium intake can rise without a lot of effort, just by not knowing what you are eating. If you enjoy salty snacks, oh boy! If you have three snacks a day, each one having one hundred mg Na, you are up to almost three hundred a day or more. A can of soda can easily contain twenty to thirty mg of sodium, and you will drink more than one a day (you know you can). There goes another way for sodium to rise.

Does drinking water contain sodium? Check it out, seniors.

Can you solve these mysteries concerning sodium?

1. Salt comes from sodium. True or False
2. Sodium is a mineral. True or False
3. There are many compounds that come from sodium. True or false
4. Too much sodium doesn't cause problem to the heart. True or False

5. Sodium doesn't cause excess fluid in the body. True or False
6. Patients on dialysis can have all the sodium they want. True or False
7. Processed food contains no sodium. True or false
8. Table salt is called sulfite. True or False
9. Sea salt and kosher salt are not really a source of sodium. True or False
10. Fresh beets are the vegetable with the lowest sodium. True or False
11. It is healthy to cook with tons of salt; just don't shake any on cooked foods. True or False
12. No sodium is needed to help the body function. True or False
13. It takes a very large amount of foods and beverages to consume 2,000 mg. True or False
14. It is all right to take medications to remove fluid from the body without your doctor's permission. True or False
15. Water is a nutrient. True of False

Read further down and your questions will be answered.

Eating foods high in sodium is dangerous. Not having the desire to eat because the food is too bland does sounds familiar. It is up to you to make your food taste good without a ton of salt. Yes, it can be done and is being done by me every meal. Friends and family are no excuse. Cardiovascular conditions are not a game of relaxed checkers or bridge (smile). Not taken care of properly it is a KILLER. Our bodies need sodium for proper body functions, and the body lets us know when there is too much or too little. Let's not ignore the messages our bodies give. Passing up a feeling of illness or even intuition that something is wrong happens to most of us; this doesn't take whatever it is away. Puffy legs and feet and shallow breathing were my warning. If you wait too long to follow why it is going on, you will be asking from a hospital bed in the cardiac unit. I was blessed, and thanks to the alertness of my medical staff, I came out a winner. This happened eight years ago, but to me it is my warning every day.

Sodium can be an enemy if not used properly. I found that my basket has become very full with health issues within a very short time, but it was long in coming. When we are young some of our responsibility to know the better side of us can be ignored. I saw it five to six days a week, but I was young, happy, and carefree. Even after being well educated in my duties, I never dreamed that I would be the patient one day. Our condition is nothing to be ashamed of; the shame is in the neglect. Some of the health illnesses that some of us share are from birth. Let us not use this fact as an excuse not to help ourselves. My parents had hypertension; this doesn't give me the excuse not to try hard to keep mine in control. Our parents lived in their time and did what was necessary to survive; this is another time. The genes we share never leave us, but the brain always has room for a better tomorrow. Thanks to new technology and science, some of us are now being helped in a better way than our loved ones were. Technology and science are awesome plusses for mankind.

H.H.S. Tip
Remember that sodium has partners in crime for those who are battling cardiovascular conditions.

Answers To Low-Sodium Questions

The following are the answers to the low-sodium questions.

1. True
2. True
3. True
4. False
5. False
6. False
7. False
8. False
9. False
10. False
11. False
12. False
13. False
14. False
15. True

If you answered the majority right, give yourself a hug.

Food Choices For Low-Sodium Meals

Correct Food Choices for Low-Sodium Meal

- Unsalted broths and soups
- Lean fresh meats and occasional seafood
- Starches low in salts and fats
- Vegetables with low-sodium counts
- Fats low in sodium and saturated fats
- Desserts: fresh fruits daily, low-sodium choices of canned fruits, and desserts. Low-fat choices ...
- Skim milk
- Juice: small low-salt vegetable juices, unsalted tomato juice, low-sodium fruit juices

Incorrect Food Choices for Low-Sodium Meal

- Soups and broths with high sodium
- Meats that have been cured and are full of fat. Too much seafood in your meal planning
- Starches high in sodium and fats
- Eating vegetables with high sodium count (such as beets too often), adding salty seasonings
- Fats high in sodium, all unhealthy fats, and cholesterol
- Desserts: pastries, pies, cakes, cookies. Ice cream and sherbets need close label and ingredient reading.
- Any type of salt is a no-no.
- Juices with added sodium with a high count
- Receive the proper advice before using any salt substitutes (put up the red light)

Be extra safe: make your own seasonings. It's easy!

Look Out When Eating Out

1. Stay away from salty condiments, ketchup, mustard, dressings.
2. Don't nibble on salty snacks.
3. Omit heavy seasoned sauces and gravies.
4. Make fruit and vegetables a part of your meals.
5. Inquire about how your food will be prepared if eating out. Ask, if you are not doing the cooking.
6. Don't indulge in an overload of fast foods when out.
7. Stay away from foods that wet your palate for salt.
8. Stay away from eating large amounts of processed foods (hot dogs, sausage, deli meats, salty soft pretzels, highly salted pizza, the cheeses and sauce that are often used) and overloading on soft drinks, ice cream, and everything else that tastes good! (smile).
9. Don't follow your eating party; follow what is needed for your meal to be healthy and enjoyable.
10. Don't let going out to eat make you forget what should be going into you.

SECTION FIVE

Combination Health Conditions Need Combination Meal Planning

There are illnesses that connect to each other. Diabetes and cardiac disease is one of the most popular combinations. Why? It appears to me that one illness can affect other organs. I started with high blood pressure, and when I looked around years later I had developed cardiac and diabetes disease. As I stated earlier in my book, this is all about me sharing my struggles with you. I am not offering anyone any medical or dietary information unless I have been involved personally with the situations; then I will discuss how it is affecting me. There are more combined diets than ever: diabetic, cardiovascular, hypertension—the listing and grouping goes on and on ... Those who don't fit in any of these categories, don't shake your heads in disbelief. Get real; it happens, and it is all around us. This type of diet takes not only good nutritional skill but patience with the patient. This diet will be around as long as there are sicknesses. Very few have one condition in their health. With good imagination from the person setting up the meal and the cooperation from the patient the meal can be a winner. It was happening since the 1960s and hopefully is still being made possible ... A good understanding of the condition and the willingness to connect both has always been a winner in my book. Know your food enemies in planning your meals, keep them out, and you will reach the gold. Healthy meals have to be thought about, and in addition making them happy is fun.

When you shop for the foods and you have a combination of red lights on, reading the food labeling is very essential.

You are looking for appropriate amounts of fats, sugar, sodium, and cholesterol. You mustn't just concentrate on the condition that may be the largest concern; all three are important.

It takes more than sugar to make glucose get out of way and more than sodium for your cardiac condition to take a turn for the worse.

The following is real and became a large part of my continued trail down a long and steep hill in the patient-care field. The following information can enlighten you as to how it really comes alive.

These are the special diets that have to be handled with compassion and a drive to do it all the best you can. Don't settle for less when it comes to your life.

Preparing a Meal for Mrs. P. and Mr. Bob

Mrs. P. has been instructed by the dietician to be on an 1,800 calorie and low-salt diet. The following is a meal that can be a guideline just for her (and you):

BREAKFAST
½ cup cereal
1 boiled egg white
½ slice wheat toast with sugar-free preserves
1 tsp unsalted soft margarine
1 cup stewed fruit
Decaf beverage

LUNCH
½ cup white and black bean turkey soup (no added salt)
Stuffed pita fresh vegetable sandwich with light dressing (mixed veggies and low-sodium, low-fat cheese)
½ cup mixed fresh and canned fruit (no added sugar)
Snack: fried apples with a garnish of fresh mint
Decaf tea with lemon and artificial sweetener
½ cup flavored skim milk
Snack: low-fat, sugar-free black and white pudding
Condiments allowed: artificial sweetener, unsalted seasonings. Use salads with precaution to avoid high-sodium veggies; make all dressings and fats low in sodium and saturated fats. Leave it to the patient as always to be sure that they can tolerate the food offered.

I conduct my meal planning for my family and myself, still using the old familiar ways. Is this meal great or what? Come on, seniorhood, we have the last of the real true knowledge of how it truly was. Give a shout for the seniorhood. Pick up my recipe book. The black and white bean turkey soup and other recipes mentioned are all there. Diabetics, high blood pressure, and cardiovascular friends, come on for a tasty, flavorful seat at my table.

Another patient in need of a special diet of 2,000 calories and low sodium and low cholesterol is Mr. Bob.

BREAKFAST
1 egg substitute/cheese omelet (1 serving eggs with 1 ounce low-salt, low-cholesterol cheese)
½ English muffin with soft unsalted margarine and sugar-free jam
½ cup applesauce
½ cup unsweetened juice
½ cup flavored skim milk
Decaf beverage with artificial sweetener

I'll leave Mr. Bob's lunch up to you.

DINNER
½ cup cream of asparagus soup (unsalted)
Baked chicken no skin and unsweetened peaches
½ cup eggplant delight (use an herbal garlic seasoning)
Small hard dough roll with unsalted margarine
Cherries jubilee (sugar free and fat free)
1 cup skim milk
Decaf beverage with artificial sweetener
Mid-afternoon snack: 1 cup air popcorn unsalted with curry flavoring; ½ cup low-sugar Jell-O
Keep vegetables in good serving sizes; eating two at one meal is okay if allowed.

Try preparing certain long-cooking foods a day or two ahead. It is great to be able to make meals just for you.

Let's continue to know what your limitations are in choosing your foods.

Dialysis Alert

Please, seniors, if you are on dialysis, please leave the salt, high-potassium foods, and overload of fluids alone. How can you eat a hot sausage with extra mustard, fries, drowning in ketchup, and thirty-two ounces of orange juice???? You are putting your life on a very narrow line.

You do know better. You have been given the rules; make a habit of following them.

Keep all the red lights on. If a renal diet is your regimen to follow, don't turn the lights off unless you are told to professionally. I used the above menu because I had seen this eaten twice by a very dear friend (a hard-headed one). I will keep talking and doing all I can to have my friend with me for as long as possible ...

An Unfamiliar Diet

I came into work one morning feeling like I SHOULD HAVE STAYED HOME. I was given a new patient with a diet I had never done a meal plan for. Oh no, not today, I thought. We all have had these days at one time or another, right? The patient had a disease called CELIAC DISEASE. I had quite a bit of education in most of the common diseases and diets, but this was not one of them. This disease calls for a gluten-free diet. Well I was working with someone who wasn't going to give any extra information; I thought I had better spend my lunchtime in the facility library. This would be good timing; the patient wasn't arriving until mid-afternoon and was coming from out of state. I had to do a good job to gain a chance for more responsibility with one-on-one patient-nutrition care. I was new, and this was a great opportunity to strut my stuff (smile).

I am glad that it was done the hard way. Learning can be hard sometimes without the support, but it will make you a much stronger person, and what you learn will stay with you for years to come.

Mr. Henry came in, and I started right away talking and getting to know him and his food likes and dislikes.

If you are not familiar with this particular condition or diet this is how it goes.

CELIAC CONDITION affects the intestines. GLUTEN is a natural protein found in some grains such as barley, wheat, rye, and oats. The body cannot tolerate these grains. Once the gluten metabolizes in the body, it becomes GLIADIN. The gliadin does the real damage to the walls of the small intestines; the walls have to stay healthy because they are the absorbers needed in order to receive the nutrients from foods. This can cause malnutrition if the absorption doesn't take place properly. Celiac disease has been determined to be a genetic disorder. I had to give Mr. Henry a meal that was the least boring possible; it had to be appetizing and nourishing and stay within his food allowances. Oh boy.

Mr. Henry's First New Meal on a Gluten-Free Diet

LUNCH
Sliced hot veal with mild gravy made with rice flour
Sliced hot green beans with garlic-flavored margarine
Fresh mashed white potatoes with gravy
Tapioca pudding with sliced peaches
Hot beverage

The patient was pleased and ready for a snack before dinner. Just a dish of sherbet was given.

DINNER
Okra, onion, and garlic soup
Lamb chop with mint jelly
Creamed beets with peppers
Decaf beverage
Canned pears
flavored milk
Snack: rice cake/fruit

This patient could not tolerate milk. He was not lactose intolerant; he had never learned to drink milk. A flavored milk was the answer to his non-milk drinking.

I showed him how drinking milk can be fun and tasty.

I sent him home with some new ways to make milk good.

There are certain things that happen in our lives that never leave; the above was mine. Just last year I met a new friend who has celiac disease, and I can understand her needs in meal planning. I help her make her grocery list. We never know what changes will take place in our lives, especially when you have a head start on certain health conditions.

Keep connecting with each other, seniors.

Learning From Errors

Most of the time, people learn from their errors. This is what most scholars consider becoming wiser and stronger in life's surprises. We stay away from what we should not do by listening to others. We can have all that life offers, in wealth, understanding, and clout with the rich and famous, gorgeous to look upon in manner and physical beauty; all this we can have, but without GOOD HEALTH being a part of it, it is zero that we have. This is a message all can take advantage of.

When we error, the next step should be the learning process. Take your errors and turn them into a better understanding and a better way to deal with any errors to come. Let's make the errors in our lives be our future strength for better and healthier tomorrows.

If we don't learn from our errors, how can knowledge and directions become more positive? Carry all your trials and tribulations in life in a tightly closed sack. When the proper time to open it arises, you'll be surprised at how those trials and tribulations in your life have become miniature.

A Mistake Is A Mistake

There should be no room for pouting, anger, or rudeness in a senior's life. Reach inside of yourselves and every day bring out the strength, determination, and all the positives that are there to be used for the good of your life. We can do this together, never even knowing each other's name.

WHY?
BECAUSE THIS WILL BE OUR LEGACY!
HOW?
BY CONNECTING IN HOW HIGH WE CARRY OUR FLAG FOR THE HEALTH OF THE SENIORHOOD

When you feel alone in your fight for health, pick up this book and join me, and let's share our struggles.

Let my recipes and meal planning book help you to fight your problems in meal planning.

Thanks, readers, for making another happy, healthy book; your book.

TAKE YOUR MEDICATIONS

EAT HEALTHY

BE HAPPY

BE A WINNER

WAVE YOUR FLAG

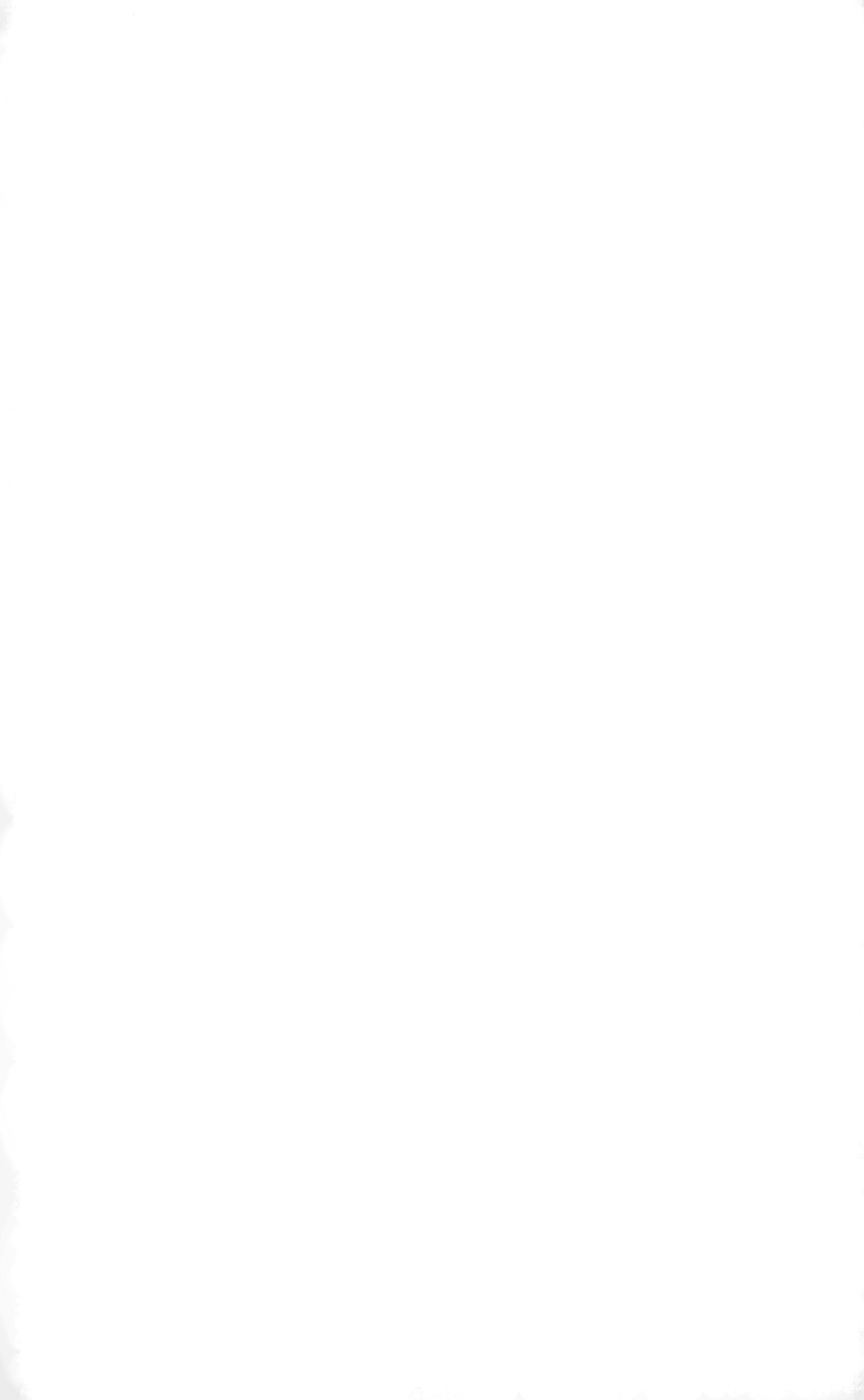